Low Fodmap Diet

Dietary Guidelines For Managing IBS, Reducing Digestive
Symptoms, And Improving Overall Health

(How To Begin The Low-Fodmap Diet With Easy Comfort
Foods)

Giandomenico Morelli

TABLE OF CONTENT

Introduction

If You Have Been Suffering From A Functional Stomach Disorder Such As Ibs And Have Been Unable To Pinpoint The Cause Of Your Symptoms, Then The Low Fodmap Diet May Be The Breakthrough You Have Been Searching For. A Low Fodmap Diet Has Assisted Numerous Individuals In Restoring Harmony To Their Gastrointestinal Framework And Relieving Them Of The Long-Term Distress And Discomfort.

This Book Provides The Fundamental Information You Need In A Straightforward, Easy-To-Follow Format, Empowering You To Assume Responsibility And Effectively Manage Your Situation.

In This Quick Start Guide, You Will Learn Which Food Sources To Avoid And

Which Food Varieties You Can Eat, As Well As How The Diet Works And How To Identify Your Triggers, Along With Numerous Helpful Tips And A Plethora Of Delicious Low Fodmap Recipes. You'll Be Able To Quickly Implement Your Healthier Eating Plan With Mouthwatering Ideas For Breakfast, Lunch, Dinner, Pastries, And Treats, So You Won't Feel Like You're Missing Out On Anything. Are You Ready For The Exam? Why Don't We Get Started?

Fodmap Is An Acronym For Fermentable Oligosaccharides, Disaccharides, Monosaccharide's, And Polyols, Which Are Regarded As Normal Triggers Found In Common Food Sources And Can Cause Stomach-Related Problems. Certain Difficult-To-Digest Starches Are Responsible For The Notoriously Unpleasant Symptoms Of Irritable Bowel Syndrome.

The low FODMAP diet was researched and developed by an Australian group at Monash University in Melbourne, led by Drs. Sue Shepherd and Peter Gibson. They observed that a low FODMAP diet, one low in food varieties containing specific sugars, was suitable for alleviating gastrointestinal symptoms in patients with IBS and other gastrointestinal symptoms. Since that time, the low FODMAP diet has spread worldwide and been adopted by dietitians and specialists as a viable method for managing stomach symptoms.

Chapter 1: The Process Of Adopting The Low-Fod Map Diet

Because it is designed to eliminate foods that may cause digestive discomfort, the low-FODMAP diet provides very little room for flexibility. If you modify the recipes to eliminate FODMAPs, you can tailor the diet to include your favourite foods, but you must adhere to the plan to be successful. If vegetarian meals, baked goods, smoothies, and even Paleo options fit your dietary needs, you can still enjoy them; simply read the ingredient lists before consuming. The low-FODMAP diet offers a variety of scrumptious, nutrient-dense meals to meet your specific dietary requirements without making you feel deprived. If you need to modify the low-FODMAP diet for medical conditions such as diabetes, your supervising dietitian can ensure that you adhere to your medical requirements.

Does the low-FODMAP diet permit weight reduction? On the low-FODMAP diet, certain foods are consumed with moderation. Such portion consciousness is an excellent place to begin when attempting to lose weight. As long as you do not severely restrict your diet, you can reduce calorie intake by adjusting portion sizes. Ensure that you are eating enough to maintain your energy and general health. On the low-FODMAP diet, many individuals report unintentional weight loss. It is difficult to determine whether this is because they are paying closer attention to what they eat or because intestinal inflammation and water retention have decreased.

Chapter 2: Searching For Fodmap Dietitians

A registered dietitian should supervise your low-FODMAP diet to ensure its nutritional integrity. Because a dietitian and a nutritionist are two distinct professions, you must ensure that you are speaking with the appropriate expert. Dietitians are qualified to provide advice on all aspects of dieting and eating, including specialised diets such as low-FODMAP. Dietitians are credentialed through accredited educational institutions, and this profession is governed. Although nutritionists are frequently unable to provide advice on specific diets, they can provide guidance on healthy eating.

Request a list of registered dietitians who can assist you with a low-FODMAP diet from your doctor or the regional hospital. If you conduct a local dietitian search on the Internet, you will find an abundance of resources. Just be sure to concentrate your search on dietitians with expertise in low-FODMAP diets.

Request a list of registered dietitians who can assist you with a low-FODMAP diet from your doctor or the regional hospital. If you conduct a local dietitian search on the Internet, you will find an abundance of resources. Just be sure to concentrate your search on dietitians with expertise in low-FODMAP diets.

Chapter 3: Low Fodmap Diet

FODMAP stands for fermentable oligo-, disaccharides-, mono-, and polyols. These are short-chain carbohydrates (sugars) that are poorly absorbed by the small intestine. The LOW FODMAP DIET is a diet low in these carbohydrate types. These particular short-chain carbohydrates are osmotically active, which means they draw water into the digestive tract without being digested.

The majority of FODMAPs are classified as indigestible forms of dietary fibre. They exit the digestive tract in the same state as when they entered. FODMAPs are generally harmless unless excessive quantities of foods containing them are consumed.

In addition, because they cannot be digested, stomach bacteria ferment them, which increases the production of gas and short-chain fatty acids.

FODMAPs have a well-deserved reputation for causing digestive symptoms such as bloating, gas, stomach pain, and constipation, diarrhoea, or a combination of the two.

More than sixty percent of individuals with irritable bowel syndrome (IBS) have indicated that these carbohydrates may cause or exacerbate their symptoms.

A variety of foods contain FODMAPs, though in varying concentrations. Some foods contain only a single type, while others contain multiple types. These foods are the most prevalent sources of each of the four types of FODMAPs:

Wheat, rye, almonds, legumes, artichokes, garlic, and onions contain oligosaccharides.

Products containing lactose, such as milk, yoghurt, soft cheese, ice cream, buttermilk, condensed milk, and whipped cream, are disaccharides.

Monosaccharides are fructose-containing foods like apples, pears, watermelons, and mango. Monosaccharides

Include sweeteners that contain fructose, such as honey, agave nectar, and high fructose corn syrup.

Mannitol and sorbitol are found in foods such as apples, pears, cauliflower, stone fruits, mushrooms, and snow peas. Xylitol and isomalt are found in low-calorie sweeteners such as sugar-free gum and mints.

The Low FODMAP Diet Consists of Three Phases

The most commonly recommended and prescribed low-FODMAP diet consists of three steps: elimination, re-challenging, and personalization.

Phase 2 : The Elimination Procedure

The first step of the low-FODMAP diet is the elimination phase, also called the restriction phase. This stage is also referred to as the restriction stage. During this phase of the treatment, you will abstain from FODMAP-rich foods for anywhere between two and six weeks. This may be the lowest rung

FODMAP procedure is the most difficult because these carbohydrates are present in many foods and are difficult to avoid.

The researchers who were the first to study the low FODMAP diet assert that the majority of online information is either inaccurate or obsolete. They stress the significance of having qualified dietitians and medical professionals.

Banana Friands

Prep time: 6 10 min| Serves: 2 2|
Difficulty: Moderate
Nutrition: Calories: 299 kcal |Fat: 2 6 g|
Protein: 2 2 g| Carbohydrates: 28 g

Ingredients
- 9 tablespoons unsalted butter, cut into cubes
- 2 2 /8 cups confectioners' sugar, plus more for dusting 2 /8 cup cornstarch
- 2 /8 cup superfine white rice flour 2 2 /8 cups almond flour
- 10 large fresh egg whites, lightly beaten
- 2 tablespoon plus 2 teaspoon fresh fresh lemon juice 2 teaspoon vanilla extract
- 2 small ripe banana, peeled and roughly chopped

Instructions

14

1. Turn the oven's temperature to 6 10 0 degrees (2 80 degrees Celsius). Lightly oil a 2 2-cup muffin pan, fry pan, or small loaf pan with cooking spray.
2. Melt the butter in a small skillet over low heat, then easy cook for 6 to 8 minutes, or until brown specks appear.
3. Take it out of the equation. Sift the rice flour, cornstarch, and confectioners' sugar three times in a large mixing basin (or whisk in the bowl until well combined).
4. Using a large metal spoon, stir in the almond flour before incorporating the fresh egg whites, fresh lemon juice, vanilla, and melted butter. Add the pieces of banana and mix thoroughly.
5. Fill each cup with the batter until they are two-thirds full. Bake for 2 2 - 2 10 minutes until firm and lightly golden (a toothpick inserted into the center should come out clean). Cool the cake in the pan for five minutes before transferring it to

a wire rack to finish cooling. Just before serving, dust with confectioners' sugar.

Pesto With Cilantro, Chile, And Mint

Ingredients

- 1 cup olive oil
- 2 tsp. sugar
- 2 tsp. salt
- 4 cups tightly packed fresh cilantro leaves
- 2 cup tightly packed fresh mint leaves
- 2 small fresh green or red chile, chopped
- 2 tbsp. minced fresh ginger
- 4 tbsp. water
- 6 tbsp. fresh lime juice 4 tbsp. walnut pieces

Directions:

1. In a food processor or blender, combine the chile, ginger, water, lime juice, walnuts, oil, sugar, and salt.

2. Blend until smooth.

3. While the blender is running, open the lid's hole and cram handfuls of cilantro and mint leaves inside; you may need to cover the lid's hole with your hand between additions of leaves to simply avoid spilling.

4. until you get a grainy paste, just keep processing.

5. If desired, freeze in little pieces or chill until ready to serve.

Carrot Muffins

just keep **Coconut oil**

- 2 large ripe banana
- 8 large fresh eggs , lightly beaten
- 2 cup grated carrots
- 2 tablespoon maple syrup
- 4 teaspoons pure vanilla extract
- 1 cup almond flour
- ½ cup coconut flour
- 2 tablespoon ground cinnamon
- 2 teaspoon ground nutmeg
- ½ teaspoon sea salt

fresh eggs

1. Preheat the oven to 350 degrees Fahrenheit. Lightly grease two regular muffin pans with coconut oil to make 20 cups.

2. In a small mixing bowl, thoroughly combine the almond flour, coconut flour, cinnamon, nutmeg, and salt.

3. 6 . Mash the banana with a fork in a medium bowl until it is a smooth purée.

4. Combine the fresh eggs , carrots, maple syrup, and vanilla in a mixing bowl.

5. Stir together the flour and banana mixture to produce a smooth batter. Fill the muffin pans to approximately three-quarters full with the batter.

6. Bake for 45 to 50 minutes, or until the muffins spring back when gently touched in the middle.

7. Allow the muffins to cool for a few minutes in the muffin pans before transferring them out onto a cooling rack.

8. Just keep muffins in an airtight container at room temperature for up to 1-5 days.

Pesto Pasta With Chicken And Tomatoes Roasted In The Oven

Ingredients:

Broiled Tomatoes

- 4 (0.710 oz.) bundles new basil
- ½ cup chives
- ½ cup pine nuts
- 1 lemon, juice of
- ½ cup garlic-mixed olive oil
- Salt and pepper, to taste
- 2 6 cherry tomatoes, split
- 2 Tbsp. garlic-mixed olive oil

Flame broiled Chicken

- 8 little chicken bosoms
- 2 Tbsp. garlic-mixed olive oil
- 2 tsp. dried oregano

21

Pasta

- 16 oz. uncooked without gluten pasta

  Pesto

Directions:

1. Preheat the stove to 350°F. Hurl cherry tomato parts with olive oil and spread equitably onto a shallow preparing container.

2. Easy cook until skins are wrinkled and marginally caramelized; around 60 minutes.

3. Put in a safe spot.

4. Preheat the tabletop flame broil. Spot chicken bosoms, olive oil, and oregano in a huge bowl and hurl to blend.

5. Flame broils chicken until done. Permit to cool marginally before cutting. Put in a safe spot.

6. Prepare pasta as indicated by bundle guidelines.

7. Meanwhile, place basil, chives, pine nuts, fresh lemon juice and olive oil in a blender.

8. Mix until smooth.

9. Once pasta is cooked, deplete and flush before coming back to pot.

10.   Add pesto to pasta and mix until pasta is well-covered.

11.   Top with cooked tomatoes and cut barbecued chicken.

12.   Season to taste with salt and pepper and serve warm.

Chicken Fritters

Ingredients:

.

- 4 tablespoons fresh basil, chopped

- .

- ½ cup mayonnaise

- .

- Olive oil

- .

- 4 teaspoons dried chives

- .

- Ground black pepper

- ½ teaspoon salt

- 2 lb ground chicken

-

- 4 fresh eggs

- .

- ½ cup all-purpose flour, gluten free

- .

- ¼ cup mozzarella cheese, grated

- .

Instructions:

1. Mix every one of the fixings in a bowl.

2. Heat up 2 tablespoon olive oil in a non-stick griddle over medium heat.

3. Measure out ½ cup every one of the wastes and add to the skillet, then, at that point, straighten a little.

4. Easy cook in bunches for 8 minutes for each side.

5. Easy Move to a plate fixed with paper towel. Serve.

Chapter 4: Are low-FODMAP foods vegetarian-friendly?

A vegetarian diet that is balanced may contain fewer FODMAPs. But if you don't eat meat, maintaining a low FODMAP diet may be more challenging.

This is because vegetarian staple plant-based proteins, such as legumes, are high in FODMAPs.

On the other hand, since they typically contain fewer FODMAPs than cooked beans, you can consume small portions of rinsed, canned legumes on a low FODMAP diet. Typically, a serving size equals a quarter-and-a-half cup (64 grams).

Other vegetarian foods that are low in FODMAPs and high in protein include tempeh, tofu, fresh eggs, quinoa, and the majority of nuts and seeds.

Chapter 5: What Occurs If Your Symptoms Do Not Improve?

The low FODMAP diet is not effective for all IBS patients. In reality, only about 36% of people receive any benefit from the diet.

Fortunately, non-dietary alternative treatments may be beneficial. If you wish to learn more about alternative options, consult your physician.

However, before abandoning the low-FODMAP diet, adhere to the following instructions.

1. Check the ingredient listing twice FODMAPs are frequently concealed in processed foods.

Onion, garlic, sorbitol, and xylitol are common allergens that can cause symptoms in minute quantities.

Consider the accuracy of your FODMAP data Online, there are numerous low-FODMAP food lists.

3. Consider other sources of stress

Diet is not the only factor that can exacerbate IBS symptoms. Stress is an additional significant factor.

No matter how well you eat, if you're under a great deal of stress, it's unlikely that your symptoms will disappear.

Who ought to follow a low-FODMAP diet?

A low-FODMAP diet is not appropriate for all individuals. According to research, unless you have been diagnosed with IBS, your diet may cause more harm than good. This is because most FODMAPs are prebiotics, which promote the growth of healthy gut bacteria. In addition, the majority of research has been conducted with adults.

29

Consequently, there is limited support for the diet of IBS children.

Diagnosing IBS

Irritable Bowel Syndrome (IBS) is not diagnosed using specific tests, unlike other medical conditions. This is because the test does not reveal any particularly revolting abnormalities in your digestive system. Everyone is affected differently by the condition, to varying degrees.

For this reason, the most important thing you can do is provide your doctor with a detailed description of your symptoms. In most cases, your primary care physician will consider prescribing IBS medication if you have been experiencing IBS-related symptoms for at least six months.

The Rome criteria is a classification system used for all functional gastrointestinal disorders, including irritable bowel syndrome. This criterion indicates that a diagnosis will be made if you have experienced abdominal pain or discomfort for at least one day per week over the course of the previous three months (on average). In addition to two or more of the other symptoms listed below:

• being relieved by passing stools

• frequent bathroom trips • a change in the consistency of your stools

To aid in a diagnosis, it may be beneficial to record your symptoms in a diary. This will assist in highlighting the frequency of your symptoms and identifying any patterns. You may use this as a reference when consulting with your physician.

Excluding Other Sondton

Many cases of IBS can be diagnosed based solely on the patient's symptoms. However, sometimes additional testing may be required to rule out other possible causes or conditions of the problem. For example, blood tests may be performed to rule out other conditions with similar symptoms, such as an infection or liver disease. Depending on the purpose of the test, it may also be necessary to provide a sample of your tool.

Chapter 6: The Advantages Of The Low-Fodmap Diet

Once you've eliminated the offending foods from your diet, you may be surprised by the rapid improvement. "As a clinician who has implemented the diet in many patients with IBS, the most rewarding experience has been seeing most patients feel better in just a few days," said Ssarlata.

Neha Shah, MPH, RD, an expert in digestive health nutrition at Stanford Health Care in San Francisco, informs her IBS patients that it can take from two to eight weeks to feel better.

"We're looking for less abdominal pain and less gas and bloating," he explained. It's troubling that you still have symptoms after following a low-FODMAP diet. In such a case, a registered dietitian may identify rotentional triggers, such as hidden FODMAPs or excessive consumption of low- or moderate-FODMAP foods, which may also trigger symptoms.

Chapter 7: Method That Facilitates The Initiation Of A Low Fodmap Diet

Before beginning the low FODMAP diet, it is essential to consult your physician to ensure that it is safe for you to do so. Your doctor will want to rule out soelas (celiac) disease, inflammatory bowel disease, Crohn's disease, and sanser as causes of your gastroenteritis.

These substances not only irritate your intestines like Irritable Bowel Syndrome (IBS), but also harm them, necessitating alternative treatments. Some of these medical conditions may be more difficult to diagnose once you've begun the low FODMAP diet.

The low FODMAP diet is a medically-recommended eating plan that can reduce digestive discomfort and help you determine which foods trigger your symptoms. Consider the diet a three-part educational experience: During the Low FODMAP Phase, also known as the Elimination Phase, you will consume low FODMAP meals to determine if high FODMAP foods are causing your digestive distress. This season should last anywhere between two and ten weeks.

The second step, known as "FODMAP reintroduction," involves slowly reintroducing high-FODMAP foods to your diet to determine which FODMAP category may be causing your symptoms. This stage is sometimes referred to as the "Challenge" stage.

Relaxing your strict Low FODMAP Diet and returning to the fodmap grains you tolerated well during the reintroduction phase constitutes the adapted fodmap diet or individualization phase. You will be able to eat a wider variety of foods and feel more comfortable eating out with friends and family without triggering your symptoms if you follow these steps.

The reduced FODMAP diet is not intended to be a permanent change in diet, but rather a short-term solution to relieve symptoms before beginning the FODMAP reintroduction diet. It is recommended that those on the FODMAP diet work with a knowledgeable FODMAP-trained dietitian and a medical professional to help them navigate the challenges.

As the benefits of the low FODMAP diet become more apparent, you may be more inclined to give it a shot.

If you are new to the low FODMAP diet or have tried it before but found it too challenging, this book is for you. to maintain let meexplain tweak have been using and have been working for me. Consider the admonition that follows as a means of getting started.

Backing

If you have even glanced at the low FODMAP diet's elimination list, you may have wondered, "Okay, so what CAN I eat?" The diet is lacking essential nutrients, making it unsustainable over the long term. Particularly, a wide variety of vitamins and minerals, such as magnesium and vitamin D, as well as a large quantity of prebiotics that help fuel probiotics for a healthier gut microbiome.

Since fructose is known to exacerbate IBS symptoms, the last thing you need is the Low FODMAP diet adding to your concerns.

The Second Pantru Ster Organization

If a student intends to begin the Low FODMAP diet, I advise that they do so gradually. To get started, you'll need to conduct a thorough pantry purge, separating the high FODMAP foods from the low FODMAP foods you may consume. This will help you become more organised and increase your knowledge of which foods are high in FODMAPS.

Preparing in advance Adhering to the low FODMAP diet while travelling can be difficult and taxing. Preparing for your meals and snacks in advance is strongly advised. This does not imply that you must prepare elaborate meals every day, but rather that you should always have the necessary ingredients on hand to prepare something tasty. If you plan ahead, your chances of succeeding will increase. Examine your pantry to determine what ingredients you have on hand, then base your weekly menu on those ingredients.

Zucchini And Potato Torte

Ingredients:

- 1/2 cup flour
- 1/2   cup grated Parmesan cheese
- 4 tablespoons olive oil
- Salt and pepper to taste

- 4 zucchini, spiralized
- 2 potato, boiled and mashed
- 2 fresh egg

Instructions:

1. Preheat oven to 350 degrees F. Grease a 10-inch cake pan with cooking spray.
2. In a large bowl, combine the zucchini, potato, egg, flour, Parmesan cheese, and olive oil. Mix well.
3. Season with salt and pepper to taste.
4. Pour mixture into the prepared cake pan.

5. Bake for 45 to 50   minutes or until golden brown.
6. Let cool in the pan for 10   minutes before slicing.

Basic Omelette Recipe

Ingredients

- 2 tsp sunflower oil
- 2 tsp butter
- 6 fresh eggs , beaten

Method

1. Season the beaten fresh egg with salt and pepper to taste.
2. Heat the oil and butter over medium-low heat in a nonstick frying pan until the butter has melted and is foaming.
3. Pour the fresh egg into the pan, then tilt the pan ever so slightly from side to side

to allow the fresh egg to wrl and evenly cover the pan's surface.

4. Allow the mixture to steep for approximately 40 seconds, then use a ratula to scrape a line through the centre.

5. Tilt the pan again to allow the fresh egg to run back into it.

6. Repeat once or twice more until the fresh egg is just about to hatch.

7. At this point, you may fill the omelette with any desired ingredients, such as grated cheese, ham, fresh herbs, sautéed mushrooms, or smoked salmon.

8. Spread the filling over the omelette's tor and fold it in half with the spatula. Slide onto a rlate to serve.

Low-Fodmap Satau Noodles With Chicken And Vegetables

Ingredients

4 pak choi, shredded

450 g tin bamboo shoots, drained

500 g/10 ½oz beansprouts

2 tsp grated fresh root ginger

600g/2 0½ oz dried rice noodles

2 lime, cut into wedges, to serve

8 tsp sesame seeds, to serve

2 tbsp olive oil

4 carrots, peeled and cut into batons

1 head broccoli, chopped into florets

2 10 0g/10 ½oz green beans, thinly sliced

800g/25 oz chicken breast, cut into strips

For The Sauce

pinch chilli flakes

4 tsp sesame oil

8 tbsp gluten-free light soy sauce

2 tbsp tamari

4 tbsp peanut butter

Method

1. Heat the oil in a wok or large wide pan over a medium–high heat.
2. Add the carrots, broccoli and green beans and stir-fry for 5-10 minutes.
3. Add the chicken and stir-fry for 5-10 minutes.
4. Add the pak choi, bamboo shoots, beansprouts and ginger and continue to stir-fry for another 5-10 minutes.
5. Meanwhile, bring a saucepan of water to the boil.
6. Add the noodles and cook for 5-10 minutes, then drain.

7. Add the noodles to the wok and stir through.
8. Whisk all of the sauce ingredients together in a bowl, along with 8 tablespoons water.
9. Add to the wok and stir to mix.
10. Serve immediately, with a wedge of lime and a sprinkling of sesame seeds.

Spaghetti With Citrus Pesto

- 1 tablespoon of lemon juice
- 1 tablespoon of maple syrup
- 4 tablespoons of extra virgin olive oil
- 250 g of gluten-free spaghetti
- Salt

- 10 basil leaves
- 1 orange
- 50 g of almonds
- 50 g of capers
- 8 anchovy fillets (optional)

PREPARATION

Wash and dry the basil leaves or, if they are not dirty, gently clean them with a damp cloth and dab them between 4 sheets of absorbent paper.

Peel the orange, remove the white filaments and put it in the blender together with the almonds, capers, anchovies basil, fresh lemon juice and maple syrup.

Blend until you get a homogeneous mixture.

Finally, slowly add the oil and continue to blend until creamy.

Put the pesto in a bowl and cover it with a drizzle of oil to prevent oxidation.

Close tightly with a lid or cling film. Just keep refrigerated until consumed.

While cooking the spaghetti, transfer the citrus

pesto to a bowl and add 5-10 tablespoons of

the pasta cooking water.

Drain the spaghetti and put them back in the

cooking pot. Season with the pesto, mix well

and serve.

Instantly Rotted, Low-Fodmap Tomato-Basil Risotto With Shrimp.

INGREDIENTS

• 2   jar Fody Foods Low FODMAP Tomato and Basil Sauce
• 4 teaspoons Fody Foods Low FODMAP Vegetable Soup Base
• 16 ounces brown rice fusilli or penne
• 2 cup shredded mozzarella cheese
Optional Garnish
• Thinly sliced basil leaves
• 4 tablespoons garlic-infused olive oil
• ¼   cup finely chopped leek leaves
• 1-5 pounds boneless, skinless chicken breasts or thighs • 5 cups water

Instructions

1. Set a 6-quart Instant Pot to the "Saute" setting.
2. Once the oil is hot, add the leek leaves. 1-5minutes, or until the leaves are bright green, fragrant, and tender.
3. Add the chicken substitute.
4. Turn frequently until the shsken is evenly browned, approximately 5-10 minutes.
5. To prevent a "Burn" message during pressure cooking, add a small amount of the measured water to the Instant Pot and scrape off any stuck-on food particles.
6. Instruct the "Saute" setting.
7. Add the remaining water, risotto, vegetable stock, and brown rice pasta to the chicken. Stir to blend.
8. Secure the lid of the Instant Pot and set the vent to "Sealing." Select "Manual" from the Instant Pot's menu.
9. Adjust the time on "High Pressure" to six minutes and relax.

10.   It takes my Instant Pot approximately 5-10 minutes to reheat before cooking. "Qusk Releae" the remaining pressure by carefully switching the vent to "Venting" and waiting until the remaining pressure pin drops.

11.   Using the dror pin, remove the lid.

12.   If your Instant Pot does not automatically switch to "Keep Just Warm" (most do), set the timer for thirty-six minutes.

13.   Stir cooked ratatouille and shsken. Add the cheese and stir once more.

14.   Initially, the sauce will appear yellow.

15.   The liquid was essential for soaking the rice, but it will continue to evaporate over time, resulting in a thinner sauce.

16.   To accomplish this, continue heating the rice and sauce on the "Keer Warm" setting for at least 12 minutes, or

until the sauce has reached the desired consistency.

17.   I typically wait 20 minutes prior to serving.

18.   Serve warm with traditional thinly sliced fresh bay leaves.

19.   Storage: Refrigerate in an airtight container for consumption within 3 hours and 45 minutes. Freezing is not advised.

Spicy Breakfast Scramble

Ingredients:

- 12 large eggs
- Pink Himalayan salt
- 4 tablespoons ghee
- Freshly ground black pepper
- 4 tablespoons heavy (whipping) cream
- 12 ounces Mexican chorizo or other spicy sausage
- 1 cup shredded cheese, like pepper Jack, divided 1 cup chopped scallions, white and green parts

Instruction:

1. In a large skillet over medium high heat, melt the ghee.

2. Add the sausage and sauté, browning for about 12 minutes, until cooked through.

3. In a medium bowl, whisk the fresh eggs until frothy.

4. Add the cream, and season with pink Himalayan salt and pepper.

5. Whisk to blend thoroughly.

6. Leaving the fat in the skillet, push the sausage to one side.

7. Add the fresh egg mixture to the other side of the skillet and heat until almost cooked through, about 6 minutes.

8. When the eggs are almost done, mix in half of the shredded cheese.

9. Mix the eggs and sausage together in the skillet.

10. Top with the remaining shredded cheese and the scallions.

11. Spoon onto two plates and serve hot.

Fresh Lemon Butterflies Made Without Fodmap

Fresh lemon

Ingredients:

1 cup of sans gluten self-rising flour Vanilla concentrate, a couple of drops only
Zest of half of a lemon, ground (for toppings)
400 grams fresh lemon curd
6 0 grams white chocolate shavings or curls 1/2 cup of margarine, mellowed 2 huge fresh eggs
1 cup of caster sugar
1 teaspoon of baking powder
fresh lemon

Procedure:

1.

   Preheat the stove to 350°F (2 80°C). Prepare cupcake tins by fixing tem with paper liners.

2. Combine relaxed spread and sugar in an enormous blending bowl.

3. Cream until light and soft, spread turns paler   in   color.

4. Add fresh eggs individually, beating the combination well later every option.

5. Set   aside.
   Mix all dry fixings together.

6. Give the blend a fast whisk. Gradually add the dry fixings to the margarine combination and blend well until uniformly   combined.

7. Fill the cupcake tins 1/2   full with the cake   batter. Bake for 35 to 40 minutes.

8. Until the tops become brilliant and an embedded toothpick comes out clean, easily   Remove from the broiler and cool on wire racks.

9. Once cooled, painstakingly remove the highest points of every cupcake, leaving a shallow opening. Slice the tops down the middle to make "wings".

10.   Fill the opening on top of the cupcakes with 2   teaspoon of fresh lemon curd.

11.   Top with white chocolate shavings or curls.

12.   Place the wings on the fresh lemon curd, confronting upwards to look like wings going to take flight.

Banana Toast

Ingredients:

- 2 ripe banana
- 1 teaspoon ground cinnamon
- 8 gluten-free sandwich bread slices

Directions:

1. Toast the bread to your desired doneness.
2. In a small bowl, mash the banana with the cinnamon and spread it on the toast.

Chapter 8: Low Fodmap Muffins With Coconut And Blueberries

Now that blueberries are in full bloom again, just one thing remains muffins. Only seven ingredients are needed to make these luscious muffins, and they can be prepared in under an hour.

In this phase of the diet, high fodmap foods are eliminated and replaced with low fodmap alternatives. The objective is to reach a baseline where you no longer experience food-related IBS symptoms. In Phase 2, you will then test each subgroup of Fodmaps individually to determine if they trigger symptoms. 2-6 weeks is a broad range and highly individual; if your symptoms have significantly improved in the first two weeks, you can proceed to Phase 2. If you continue to experience cramps, gas, bloating, etc., adhere to the diet until your symptoms have diminished substantially.

So, what foods are allowed on the Low Fodmap diet? - This was one of the most difficult concepts for me to grasp, as it appeared that every piece of online information contradicted one another. Some websites said I could eat avocado, while others said I couldn't. Some food lists stated that mushrooms were not permitted, but I discovered "low fodmap recipes" that included mushrooms. I was so perplexed.

The creators of the Low Fodmap Diet can provide you with accurate information regarding which foods you can and cannot eat. The Monash University Low FODMAP Diet App is an easy-to-follow guide that lists all the foods you can and cannot eat, as well as the appropriate serving sizes. This is a lifesaver - if you are at the grocery store and want to buy purple cabbage, for example, but are unsure if you can eat it, simply open the app, search for purple cabbage, and it will provide you with the necessary information. (Just so you know, a low Fodmap portion can weigh up to 7,510 grammes.)

The application includes tutorials on how to use it and additional information on the low Fodmap diet. It truly is a useful resource to possess. Currently, the price is $7.99 (Australian dollars). There are a few recipes, but sadly not many vegan options; however, the soup is delicious. I find recipes online and modify them to my liking. This will require some trial and error, but you'll quickly get the hang of it. Learning to prepare simple dishes without garlic or onions is difficult, but garlic oil can be used to add flavour, which is a plus.

To get you started, I've included a meal builder with only low-Fodmap or Fodmap-free ingredients. Choose a protein, a carbohydrate, a few vegetables or salads, and a flavour enhancer, and you're done! This can also be used to plan meals. Consult online resources to compile a list of go-to recipes and sauces, and use the App to help you create delicious dishes.

Delicious Sweet Rice Congee

- 4 tbsp cooking rice wine
- 2 cup shredded carrots
- 8 tsp freshly grated ginger
- 4 cup chopped spinach
- 1/2 tsp ground white pepper
- 4 tsp salt or to taste
- 4 tsp sesame oil
- 6 tbsp chopped green onion
- 2 cup sweet glutinous rice
- 20 cup chicken bone broth (see note below)
- 2 cup chicken liver
- 4 tsp naturally-brewed tamari soy sauce

inse the sweet glutinous rice in cold water. In a large saucepan, combine the rice and the chicken bone broth.

Easy cook for 20 minutes at a low simmer with intermittent stirring, then remove from the heat.

In the meanwhile, cut the chicken liver into tiny pieces and marinate it for 6 0 minutes in tamari and cooking wine.

Grate the ginger finely, shred the carrots, and combine them with the half-cooked sweet rice in a saucepan. Continue to easy cook for another 20 minutes.

Make tiny pieces of spinach and green onion.

Stir the spinach into the congee after adding the marinated chicken liver. Season with salt and freshly ground white pepper to taste. Easy cook for a further 2 0 minutes.

Toss in sesame oil and remove from heat when done. As desired, garnish with green onions.

Chapter 9: Tips For Implementation

In daily life, it is not always simple to strictly adhere to a list of acceptable food sources. Whether it is a business dinner, a gathering with friends, or a family outing to a café, dining out is a common occurrence. Initially, only one out of every odd restaurant has acceptable dishes that FODMAP-reduced acquaintances may enjoy. It means eating regimen for you. Even acquaintances and you must design a great deal in order to know which foods are acceptable, particularly at the beginning of your diet change. This piece can be depleting in the beginning. But do not let this depress you. You will quickly become accustomed to your new diet and will soon be able to deal with it routinely and without stress.

Obviously, you can inform your family in advance which food sources you can tolerate and which you cannot. Assuming that your companions are somewhat perplexed, you can send them a couple of recipe suggestions to ensure that nothing disrupts the general flow of a pleasant dinner together. Perhaps you should first invite your loved ones to your home and prepare a divine meal. Thus, you can persuade everyone that FODMAP-friendly dinners are also incredibly delicious, given that generally uninvolved individuals have a few reservations about trying new foods. You will see, however, that the others will be quickly persuaded that this type of diet also offers delicious meals.

The situation may become more difficult in the restaurant. Assuming you sit in a café and peruse the menu for the third time in search of dishes that are suitable for you, this can quickly become awkward and stressful. You should be able to enjoy a meal at the restaurant without having to search for a suitable dish. Currently, the majority of menus are also accessible online. Therefore, investigate the menu at home in order to avoid unnecessary pressure in the café. You may have successfully located something and can now casually anticipate your visit to the restaurant. If you haven't found what you're looking for, call the restaurant and briefly explain your issue. For what the culinary expert can provide or prepare based on your preferred food types. You can also send a brief email if you intend to visit a restaurant a few days later. In an ideal situation, you should share all food sources that you can tolerate well and that the easy cook can use to create an exceptional dish for you. Generally, restaurants will come to you and serve you a prearranged meal or two. Later, simply let us know which day you will be visiting so the easy cook can be adequately prepared.

There are certainly cafés that are more understanding of your situation than others. It is advisable to keep track of all cafés and your involvement in relation to them. Assuming you have a business lunch or dinner with friends, you have a list of restaurants from which you can choose. Your coworker has no idea why you're recommending one of these restaurants so that a terrible situation does not occur. Your companions will be pleased that you can finally return to a restaurant for a casual dinner with minimal difficulty.

In the private sector, it is advantageous if, prior to going out to shop, you carefully consider which meals you will need to prepare at home within the next few days. After deciding on all of the appropriate dishes, you should maintain a shopping list. This prevents you from remaining in the store without knowing precisely which food sources you are allowed to consume. In addition, you go shopping with a list and avoid temptations that could derail your diet. Using this method, you can additionally prevent unnecessary extras from becoming trash. Assuming you plan ahead, you can prepare meals for the following days so that you can consume all the food.

Miso Salmon

Ingredients

- 2 tsp pure maple syrup 10 g
- 1 tsp Gourmend garlic scape powder 0.6 g
- Salt and pepper, to taste

- 2 large piece salmon, or 6 small fillets if preferred 8 10 0 g
- 5 Tbsp miso paste 28 g
- 1/2   Tbsp rice vinegar 30 g
- 4 tsp soy sauce 20 g

Method

1. Season your salmon with salt and pepper. Mix the mo rate, rse vinegar, soy sauce, maple syrup, and garlic scape rowder together, and then rub the mixture all over the fish. Depending on the size of your piece(s), you may not require the entire quantity of mixture. Just gave the salmon a thin, uniform coating.

2. Preheat the oven to 4800°F (200°C), line a rimmed baking sheet with foil, and place a wire rack on the middle rack. This method will help to evenly distribute the heat in your oven throughout the food as it cooks. Place the fillets on the wire rack of the oven.

Cooking for 12 should take 510 minutes and 20 seconds. Check the temperature of the food with an instant-read thermometer; dinner is ready when it registers approximately 123.6 °F (510 °C). Do not consume food. thermometer? Simply press down gently on the top of the fillet with a fork or your finger; if the laurel leaves separate along the white lines around the fillet, it's done.

4. Remove fish from oven and allow to rest for 510 minutes prior to serving. Feel free to sprinkle lime juice and/or cilantro on tor as garnish. Serve over brown or white rice with a vegetable low in FODMAPs and enjoy!

Gluten-Free Moo Shu Vegetables

Ingredients
- 2 red bell pepper thinly sliced
- 2 orange or yellow pepper thinly sliced
- 6 cups finely shredded green cabbage
- 12 dried shiitake mushrooms rehydrated and thinly sliced (see note, optional)
- 4 scallions green parts only, julienned
- 22 Gluten-free mandarin pancakes or cassava/almond flour tortillas for serving (see note)
- 4 tablespoons gluten-free tamari
- 4 tablespoons gluten-free hoisin sauce see note, optional, plus more for serving
- 4 tablespoons Shaoxing wine sherry, sake or mirin
- 2 teaspoon sesame oil
- 1 teaspoon salt

- 6 tablespoons neutral oil I use avocado oil
- 4 medium carrots julienned

Instructions

1. In a medium mixing bowl, whisk together the tamari, hoisin sauce, wine, sesame oil, and salt. Set aside.
2. Heat a wok or large skillet over high heat.
3. Add 2 tablespoon of oil and stir-fry the julienned carrots for 1-5 minutes, until softer but still crunchy, then transfer to a bowl and set aside.
4. Using the same method, cook the red bell peppers, cabbage and shiitake mushrooms separately, and set those aside in the same bowl.
5. Be careful not to overeasy cook the vegetables – they should be pliable but still al dente.
6. Return all the vegetables to the pan and add in the sauce mixture.
7. Stir-fry everything together for another minute.

8. Serve immediately with the scallions, steamed gluten-free pancakes and more hoisin sauce on the side!

Low Fodmap Pumpkin Noodle Soup

- 1/2 tsp cayenne pepper
- A small handful of fresh cilantro
- A splash of lemon juice
- 3 stalk of spring onion
- 4 tbsp tandoori spices (make sure no low FODMAP ingredients have been added. The mix that I used contained: paprika, cilantro, salt, cumin, pepper, ginger, chilli, cinnamon and laurel)
- 1 tbsp fresh ginger
- 1 tsp turmeric
- 1 tsp ground cloves

FOR THE SOUP

- 250 g (10 .6 oz) oyster mushrooms
- 2 tbsp brown sugar
- 250 g (10 .6 oz) gluten-free noodles
- Fresh basil
- Unsalted peanuts
- 400 ml (6.7 oz) coconut milk
- 1500 ml (6 .2 cups) stock (use a low FODMAP stock cube)
- 800 g (2 8 .2) oz pumpkin in cubes
- 2 tsp fish sauce (leave this out to make the recipe vegan)

INSTRUCTIONS

1. Cut the ginger, cilantro and spring onion into very small pieces.
2. Put those together with all the spices and a splash of fresh lemon juice in a bowl.
3. Make this into a paste using a hand blender.
4. Boil the pumpkin cubes in a pan with boiling water for 20 minutes. Drain them well and use a hand mixer to make a pumpkin puree.
5. Heat some oil in a soup pan and add the spice paste.
6. Fry this for two minutes while you stir now and then.
7. Add the pumpkin puree, fish sauce and 1200 ml stock.
8. Scrub the oyster mushrooms clean, cut them into pieces and add them together with the sugar and a pinch of salt to the soup.

9. Bring the soup to a boil and leave to boil for about 20 minutes.

10. Boil the noodles according to the instruction on the package.

11. Drain them and rinse them with cold water, so they don't stick.

12. Add, after 20 minutes of cooking, the rest of the stock and the coconut milk.

13. Leave the soup to boil for another 10 minutes.

14. Add some fresh basil and the noodles to the soup and stir together.

15. Turn off the heat and leave the soup to rest for 10 minutes with the lid on the pan.

16. Serve the soup with some extra basil and chopped peanuts.

Immune Boosting Smoothie

INGREDIENTS:

- ⅛ Tsp. iodized salt
- 4 medium cucumber
- 4 tbsp. lime juice
- 4 cups ice
- 4 cups spinach
- 2 -inch ginger root, peeled
- 4 kale leaves
- 4 medium rib celery

DIRECTIONS:

1. Thoroughly rinse spinach, celery, and kale, then shake to remove any extra water.

2. Remove the tough ends of the kale and discard.
3. Scrub cucumbers well and chop into small sections.
4. Use a food blender to pulse salt, lime juice, ginger, cucumbers, celery, kale, and spinach until a smooth consistency.
5. Combine ice and continue to pulse until it reaches your desired consistency.
6. Distribute to two glasses and enjoy it immediately!

Fish And Chips Prepared With Tartar Sauce

Ingredients

- grated zest and juice 2 fresh lemon
- small handful of parsley leaves, chopped
- 2 tbsp capers, chopped
- 4 heaped tbsp 0% Greek yogurt
- fresh lemon wedge, to serve

- 900g potatoes, peeled and cut into chips
- 2 tbsp olive oil, plus a little extra for brushing
- 4 white fish fillets about 500 oz each

Method

1. Heat oven to 200C/fan 2 80C/gas 6. Toss chips in oil.
2. Spread over a baking sheet in an even layer, bake for 80 mins until browned and crisp.
3. Put the fish in a shallow dish, brush lightly with oil, salt and pepper.
4. Sprinkle with half the fresh lemon juice, bake for 25 to 30 mins.
5. After 20 mins sprinkle over a little parsley and fresh lemon zest to finish cooking.
6. Meanwhile, mix the capers, yogurt, remaining parsley and fresh lemon juice together, set aside and season if you wish.

7. To serve, divide the chips between plates, lift the fish onto the plates and serve with a spoonful of yogurt mix.

Quorn Curry Accompanied By Cauliflower Rice

- 1000 grams of frozen chicken-style Quorn or 8 00 grams of chicken chopped into pieces.
- 2 tbsp olive or avocado oil
- 4 strips of baby Pak Choy
- 200g asparagus sliced into big chunks
- 200 grams of mushrooms, sliced
- 4 spring onions, finely minced
- 2 lemongrass stem and a handful of chopped coriander leaves
- 2 small onion, chopped 2 cloves of garlic, crushed 2cm piece of root ginger, grated
- 2 tablespoon of honey
- 2 tbsp coconut aminos
- 2 tablespoon fish sauce
- 1 grain turmeric
- 2 tsp garam masala

- 800ml can of coconut milk

To Prepare Cauliflower Rice:

- optional 2 tsp coconut amino acids
- Sea salt with black pepper
- 2 cauliflower
- 2 tablespoon olive oil

1. Blend until smooth the lemongrass, coriander, onion, garlic, ginger, honey, garlic, coconut aminos, fish sauce, garam masala, and coconut milk.

2. If you have the time, marinate the Quorn or chicken for 2 hour or overnight.

3. Warm the oil in a deep skillet. Add the chicken or tofu, reserving the marinade, and stir-fry for 6 to 10 minutes.

4. Add the marinade to the remaining ingredients and simmer until the

chicken is cooked approximately 20 to 30 minutes.

5. Prepare the cauliflower rice in the interim.

6. Place cauliflower florets in a food processor and pulse until the texture resembles rice.

7. In a large skillet, heat the oil and sauté the cauliflower with coconut aminos for 5 to 10 minutes.

8. Place on plates or bowls, then cover with curry.

9. To serve, strew with spring onions.

Zucchini Carpaccio With Pine Nuts And Crisp Prosciutto

Ingredients

- 16 ounces zucchini (2 medium)

- 16 ounces summer squash Sea salt
- 6 ounces prosciutto di Parma (about 6 slices)

- ½ cup pine nuts

- ½ cup freshly squeezed fresh lemon juice
- ½ cup extra-virgin olive oil

  10 ounces baby arugula
Instructions

1. Preheat the oven to 350 °F. Line a baking sheet with parchment paper.

2. Arrange the prosciutto on the prepared baking sheet.

3. Transfer to the oven and easy cook until dark and crispy, about 20 minutes.

4. Allow to cool on the pan and break apart with your fingers into large pieces.

5. While the prosciutto cooks, toast the pine nuts: arrange the nuts in a small skillet and cook over medium-low heat until golden brown and fragrant, about 10 minutes.

6. Prep the zucchini and squash: with a sharp knife, slice as thinly as you can into rounds.

7. Arrange the zucchini and squash on a large platter, fanning out the rounds as much as possible and alternating sections of color.

8. Season lightly with salt.

9. In a small bowl or a jar with a lid, combine the fresh lemon juice, olive oil, and 1 teaspoon of salt. Stir or shake until well mixed.

10. Pour half of the dressing evenly over the zucchini and squash.

11. In a large bowl, toss the arugula with the remaining dressing and pile on top of the squash coins.

12. Garnish with the pine nuts and flecks of crispy prosciutto.

Coconut Bananas

Ingredients:

2 tsp of coconut extract

4 tbsp of agave syrup

½ tsp of cinnamon

4 large bananas, sliced lengthwise

2 cup of coconut milk

2 tsp of coconut oil

Preparation:

13.   Pour 2 cup of coconut milk in a small saucepan.

14.   Bring it to boil and stir in coconut oil, coconut extract and agave syrup.

15.   Easy cook for one minute and remove from the heat.

16.   Allow it to cool for a while.

17.   Pour this mixture on each banana slice and sprinkle with some cinnamon. Serve cold.

Fody's Low Fodmap Lasagna Zucchini Boats

Ingredients:

2 Tbsp Fody's Garlic Infused Olive Oil
4 cups Fody's Vegan Bolognese Sauce
2 1 cup shredded mozzarella
Salt & pepper, to taste
4 small zucchinis
1 cup ricotta
½ cup shredded parmesan
6 cups spinach
1/2 cup fresh basil, sliced

Directions

1. Preheat the oven to 450 degrees and line a baking dish with non-stick aluminium foil.
2. Next, remove the ends from your zucchinis and cut each one in half.

3. Use a roon to smooth out the edges, leaving a 14-inch border of zusshuni on the sides.
4. Place your zuchinni on the dish and brush them with your olive oil before allowing them to dry.
5. Then, combine your risotto, parmesan, and fresh basil in a bowl and season with salt and pepper to taste.
6. Spread a small amount of your cheese mixture on each half of the zucchini.
7. Next, chop the sage, place it in a bowl, and let it sit for a few minutes until it begins to wilt.
8. Divide the rnash evenly between your zusshn halves.
9. Pour our vegan bolognese sauce over each zucchini and pour aluminium foil over the sauce.
10.   Then, place your dough in the oven and bake for 50-90 seconds.

11.   After the pasta is cooked, flip it over and sprinkle mozzarella over the top.

12.   Place the blini in the oven and bake for 10 minutes, or until the cheese has melted.

13.   Serve medatelu and savour your Low FODMAP plant-based meal!

www.ingramcontent.com/pod-product-compliance
Lightning Source LLC
Chambersburg PA
CBHW070525030426
42337CB00016B/2107